D1732650

BETTY BOOP™
99 Secrets

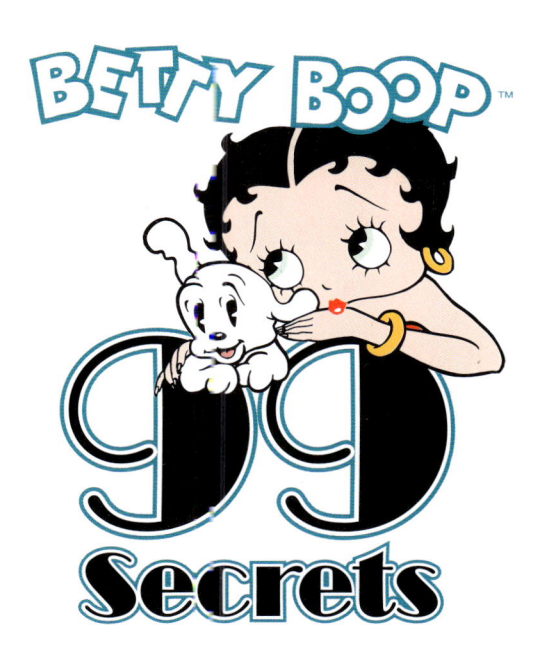

Copyright © 2010 King Features Syndicate, Inc./Fleischer Studios, Inc.
™Hearst Holdings, Inc./Fleischer Studios, Inc.

First published in 2010 by Blue Sky Books Ltd
2nd Floor, Berkeley Square House, Berkeley Square, London W1J 6BD
www.blueskybooks.co.uk

British Cataloguing-in-Publication Data:
A catalogue record of this book is available from the British Library.

ISBN 978-1-907309-01-4

Designed by Spirit Design Consultants, London
www.spirit-design.com

Editorial contribution: Sacha Markin

Printed and bound in China through Printworks Int. Ltd.

All rights reserved. No part of this publication may be reproduced, stored
in a retrieval system, or transmitted in any form, or by any means, electronic,
mechanical, photocopying, recording, or otherwise, without the prior written
permission of the publisher.

This book is intended to give general information only. The publishers expressly
disclaim all liability to any person arising directly or indirectly from the use of,
or for any errors or omissions in, the information of this book. The adoption
and application for the information in this book is at the reader's discretion and
is his or her sole responsibility.

The secret's out –
   Betty Boop
      shares all!

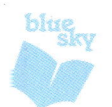

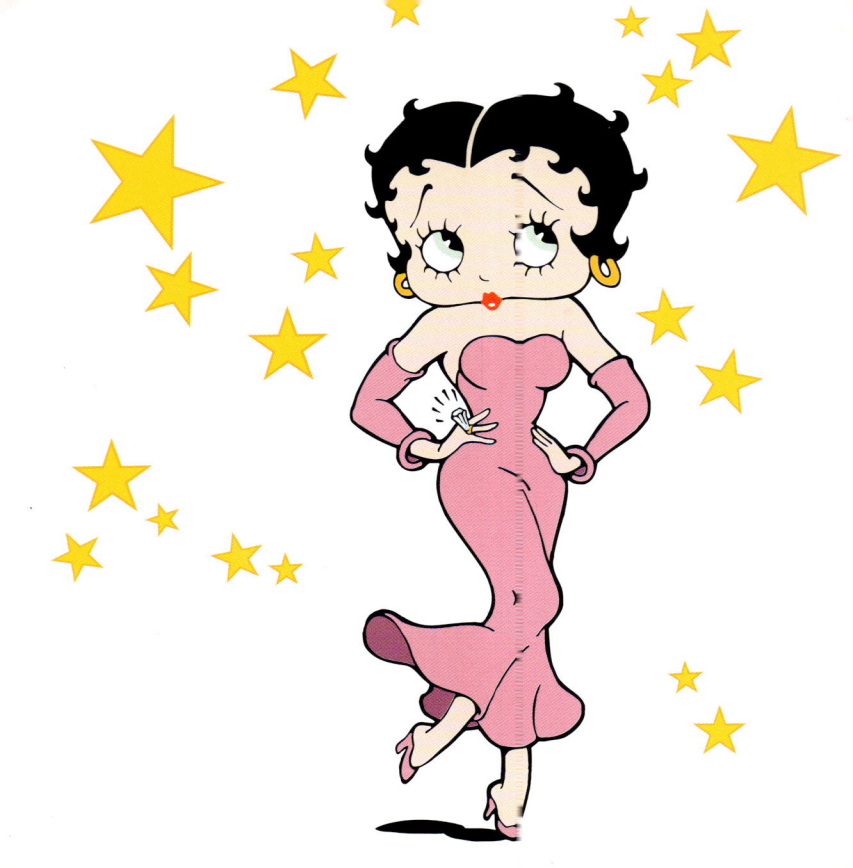

Golden Rule No 1 – Never, ever be too busy to be beautiful... never, ever, ever... promise?

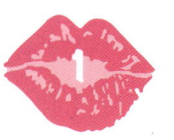

Beauty comes from inside.
Be happy! – Boop-oop-a-doop.

N-A-I-L A-L-E-R-T – your nails
are not staple removers – stop
that now!

So you've found your perfect hairdresser – never let him go! Get back here now.

Oh, pardon me, I didn't know you were watching, shaped brows always make your face looked groomed, it's a beauty fact!

Never forget your face cream – day and night!

1

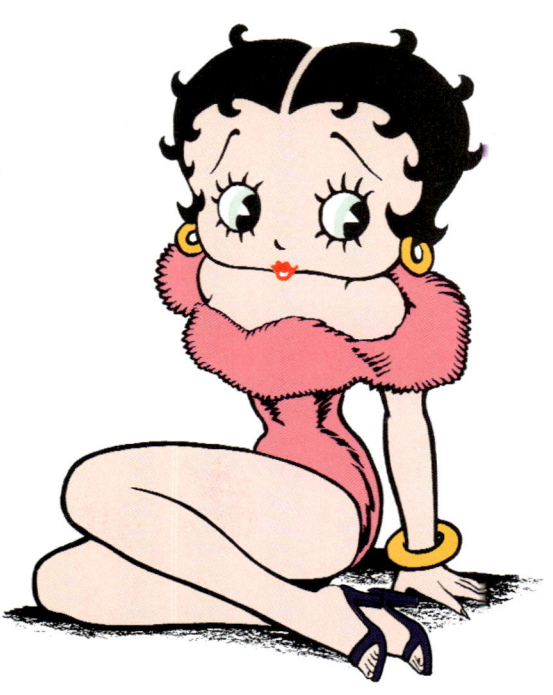

Say goodbye to bad hair days... pin it up, try a ponytail or a cute little hat... hair to go please!

Summer's here... Oh, time to switch my foundation for a little tinted moisturiser, you should try it, it's lghter and brighter. Why, you're positively glowing.

Have your dentist clean your teeth regularly – they'L feel so fresh.

For yummy summer eyes, swop black mascara for brown... that's better, wink, wink!

10

Excuse me please, where's the powder room? Treat your hair to a quick lift with warm air from the dryer – good as new.

11

Please keep all those hairbrushes and combs squeaky clean – I'll check!

12

13 Mmmmm, oh this is my favourite. Natural yoghurt makes the perfect face mask and its soooo quick and easy.

Don't run for cover sweetie, just try dabbing a little foundation under those eyes, around your nose and over cheeks. Perfect. **14**

Flutterly fabulous – curl your lashes for extra glitz – oh, you're making me blush.

All change… go from day to night by dotting a little shimmer on your face, body and hair. Boop Magic

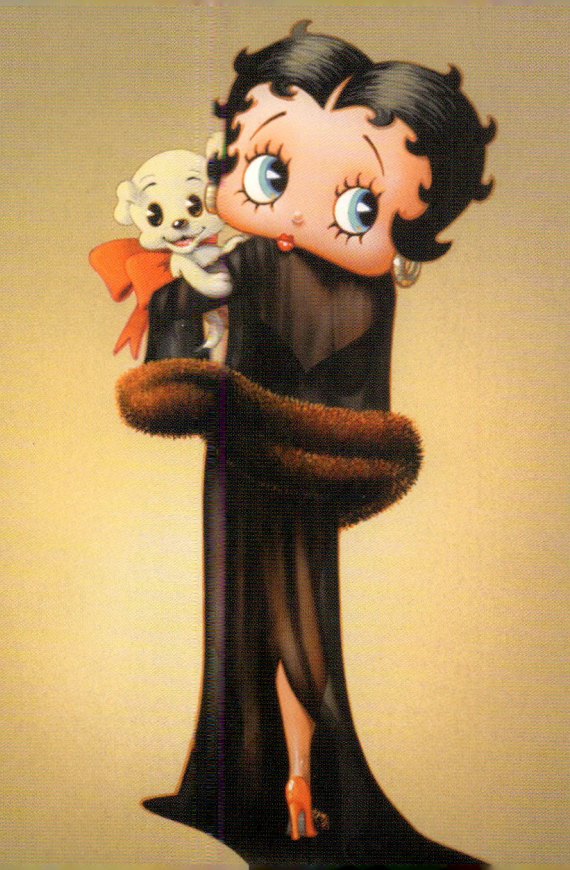

17 Stay cool... carry a little spritzer mist in your handbag. Squirt, squirt – stop that!

18 Want a Billion Dollar Face Mask? Mix a soft banana with a little honey, pat on your face and leave for 20 minutes. Wash away with warm water for heavenly skin. BOOP-LICIOUS!

And where do you think you're going? Dusting a little sheer face powder helps keeps your make-up in place, for hours and hours. Does that mean I can stay out all day?

Silk pillowcases are perfect if you've got dry hair, or curly hair, or long hair... everyone loves silk.

21

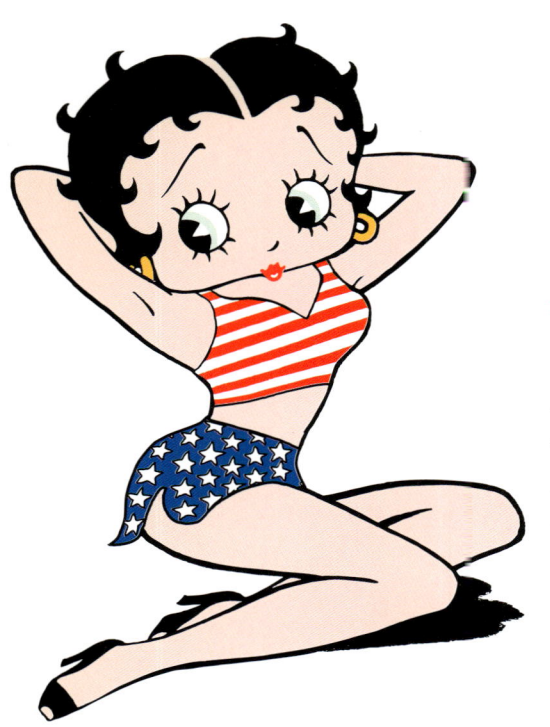

Play up your best bits, they're what Mother Nature gave you.

22 Bad hair day? Please don't cry. Try a few sparkly hair clips or clasps, there, there... that's better.

23 My face cream soaks in so much better when my face is still moist, try it, it works – ohhh that tingles

24 F-L-I-R-T A-L-E-R-T... false lashes always get results. Flutterly gorgeous!

25 Make up to go... lip-gloss, concealer and mascara – t's so simple when you know how!

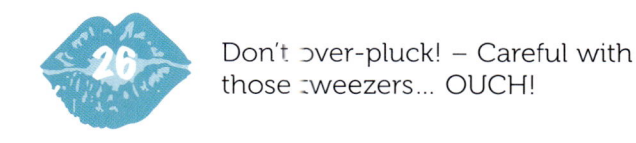

26\. Don't over-pluck! – Careful with those tweezers... OUCH!

27\. A little slice of cucumber works wonders for tired eyes... ahhh, B-L-I-S-S.

28 Get up close and personal... to a good mirror that is! Always put your eye make-up on in a good light. Ah pretty as a picture!

29 Razzle-dazzle 'em with a little highlighter below your brow... who can resist?

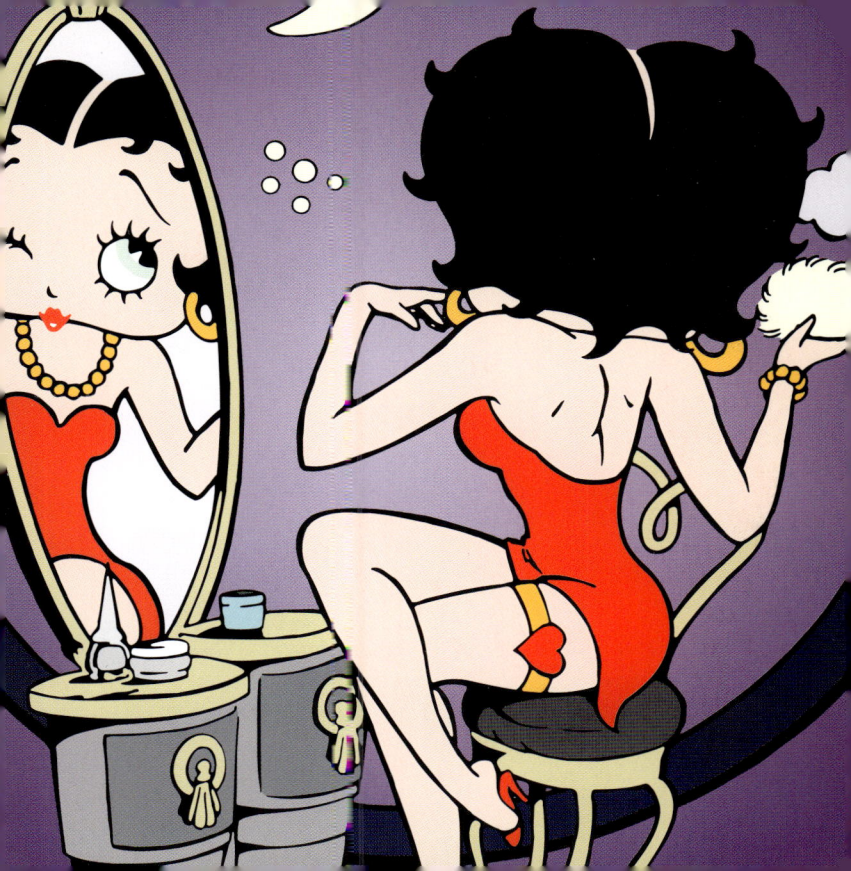

Be very, very gentle with those peepers... dot on eye cream with your itsy teeny finger... there you go! **30**

31 Make-up past its sell-by date – throw it out, throw it out!

For eyes that sparkle, white pencil below your lash line is the only way to go... lovely. **32**

33 Tired eyes, no Sirrie... dot a little highlighter on your lids for that fresh as a daisy look.

34 Hollywood here I come – for the movie star look, sweep dark eye shadow in the corner of your eyes – can I have an Oscar please?

35

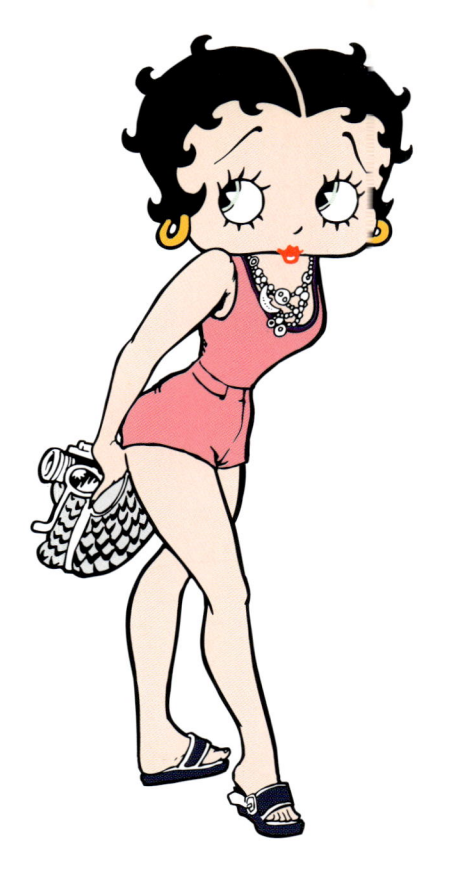

Shoulders back for
instant glamour –
slouching is a big
no, no!

36 Why you are fruity... keep those lips looking soft and lovely... dab on cherry lip gloss with your fingertips – kiss, kiss, kiss.

So you want shiny, silky hair, then rinse it quickly in cold water after washing – lovely! **37**

38 For round the clock fragrance, start with a perfume bubble bath, then body lotion and finish with a spritz of scent. 24/7 heaven!

39 Please don't sizzle those lovely locks. Dab away all moisture before blow-drying – your hair will thank you for it.

40 This is one of my very top secrets – brows should always start over the inner corner of your eye. P-e-r-f-e-c-t

41 Jeepers creepers, where did you get those peepers? Keep your eyes looking pretty; they're the first thing people notice. Flutter, flutter.

42 Safe bronzing is the only way to go... don't forget allover sunscreen for your skin...

43 Sunscreen for your hair is also a must... that's right!

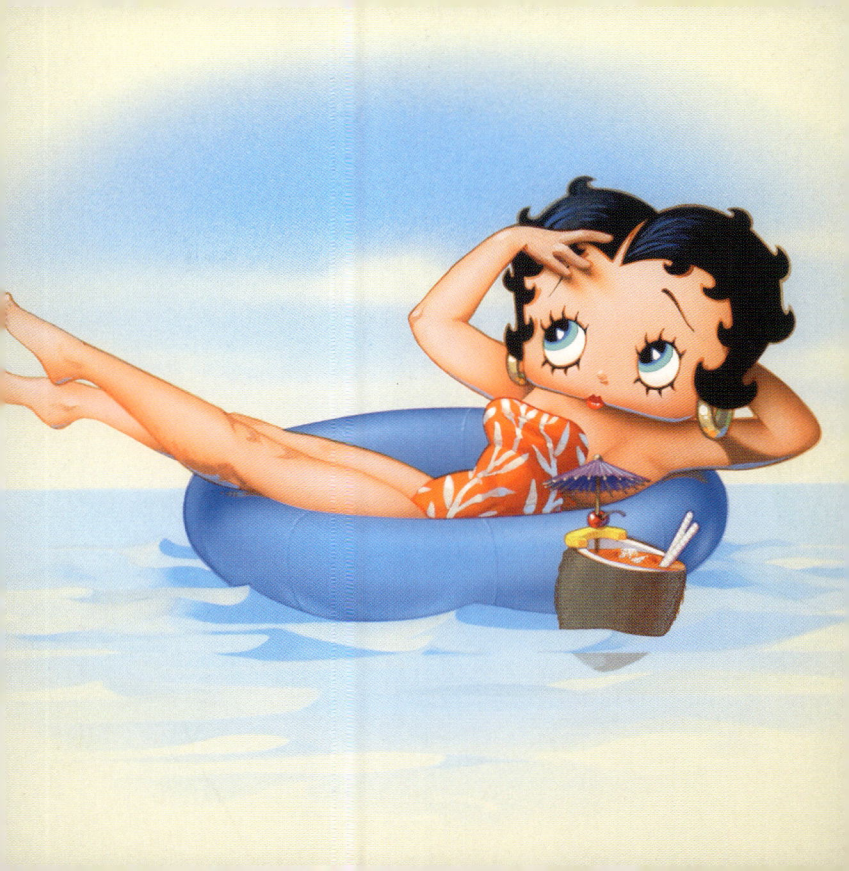

Double agent – a creamy blush also makes the perfect lipstick – twice as nice. **44**

You push your make-up bag round on wheels, it really is time to downsize – clear it out now. **45**

Lovely luscious lips and lashings of gloss – a match made in heaven. **46**

47 In a rush? Keep your nails looking good by colouring the inside with a white pencil – I told you, they look like new.

48 Your eyeliner's all squashed, oh, no... pop it in the freezer, then sharpen. I told you I was more than a pretty face.

49

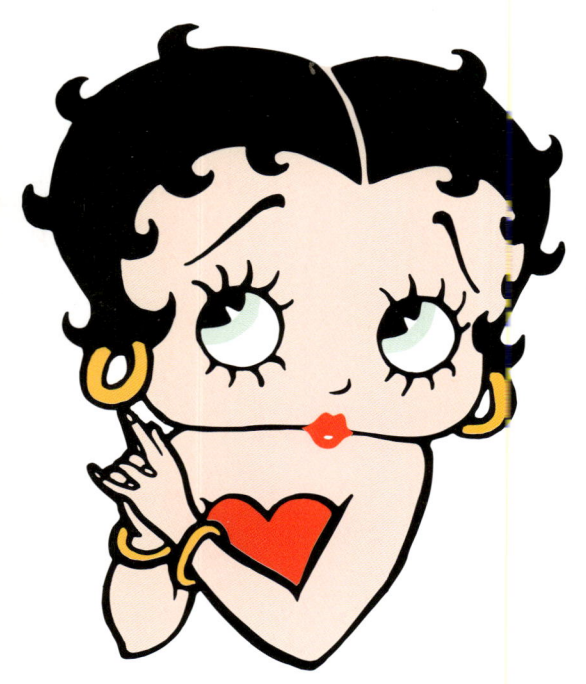

Lipstick on his
collar? No way.
Dab on a little lip
base before putting
on your lipstick.
Sweetie, this pout
is here to stay.

50 For the perfect shimmer pout, dot highlighter in the centre of your lips... lovely!

51 B-E-A-U-T-Y N-E-W-S F-L-A-S-H – take that make-up off before bed... thank you!

52 Browbeaten? You? I don't believe it – dab on clear mascara to keeps brows sleek and in-line. That's better.

53 EYECATCHING! Wearing bright colours on your eyes is fun: the secret – shhhhh – it's all in the blending, watch me!

54 All change – colouring your hair for the first time? Why not start with a wash-in wash-out – it's safer – oh, is that me?

55 Lip Service – use a liner to line and colour your lips – anything that saves time works for me.

56 Floss, floss, floss – I know, sweetie, but trust me it works!

57 Red lipstick always stops them in their tracks, (oh, I'm sorry; I think you were headed that way!) – find one that's perfect for you!

58 Go the manicure distance – touch up with clear polish every few days. I can do that.

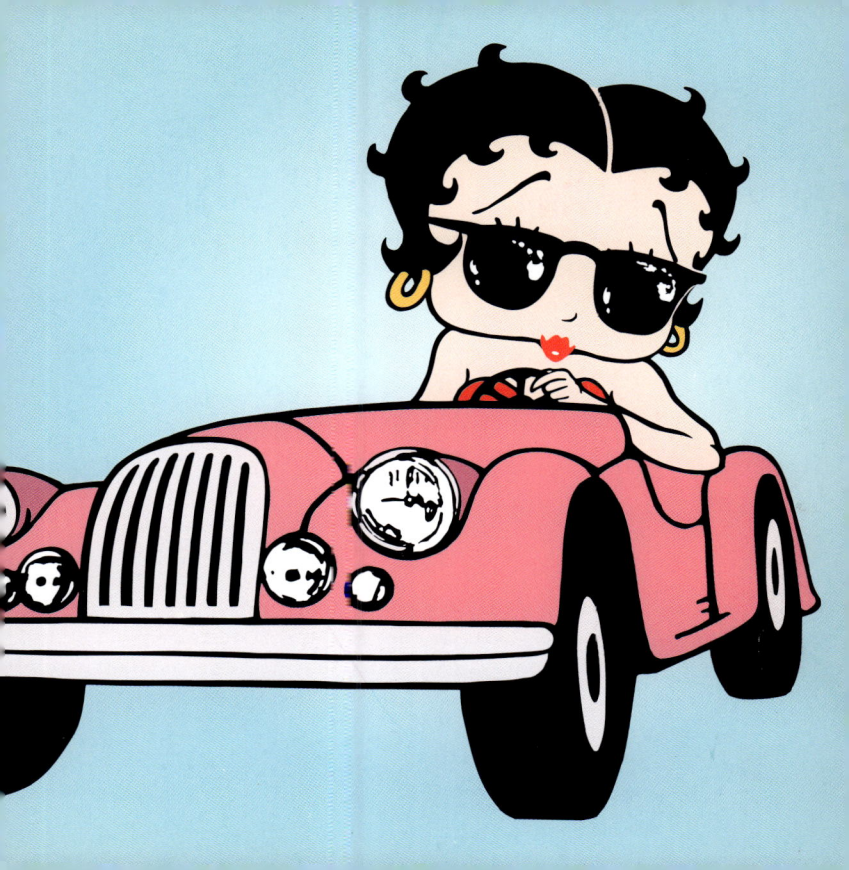

Please, please make sure your foundation is the right colour for you. Check it out in a good light on your jaw line. No excuses, please. **59**

60 A clean sweep ladies, please keep those make-up brushes clean and tidy. Thank you.

Don't forget to cleanse that lovely neck, it wants to be in on the act too! **61**

To keep you teeth pearly white, use a straw to sip your juice or coffee – that's it!

Eeny, meeney, miney, mo... Big eyes, natural lips or natural eyes, big lips? Only one please.

64

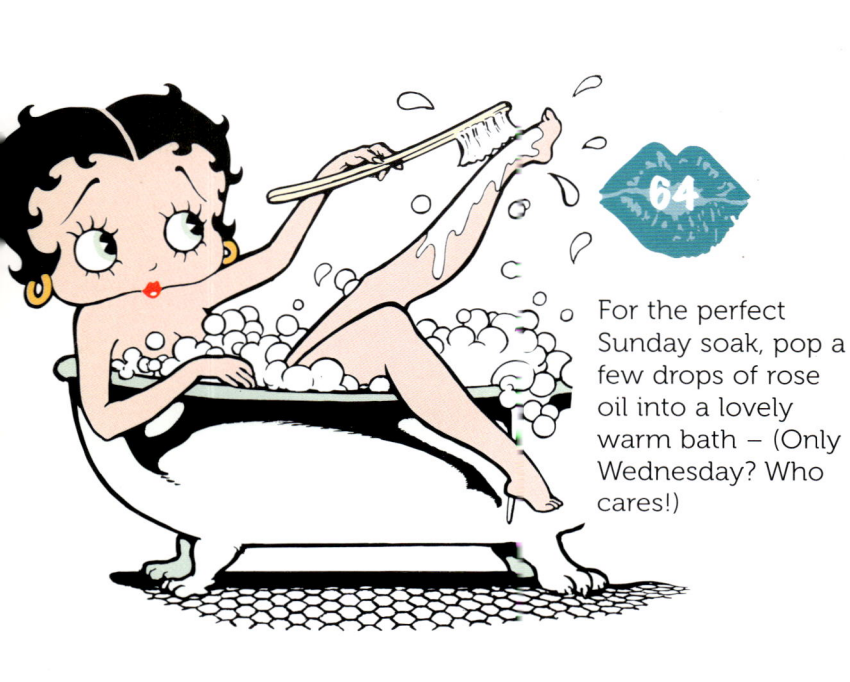

For the perfect Sunday soak, pop a few drops of rose oil into a lovely warm bath – (Only Wednesday? Who cares!)

So you want perfect evening lips? Use a lipstick one or two shades lighter or darker than your daytime one – what do you mean you hardly recognised me – boop-oop-a-doop!

Go easy on the foundation; you don't want to scare them.

67 Away with you – zap away those naughty blemishes with a dab of tea-tree oil at bedtime. Thank you; now please do not come back!

68 Do you have a license for those lashes? Layer on lashings of mascara, for eyes that say... hello there!

Moisturise, moisturise, moisturise! You want soft, silky skin, don't you? **69**

70 Dab a little highlighter on your shoulders and neck line for extra glamour. Boop-oop-a-doop!

Why you cheeky little thing, you want instant colour, then sweep some rosy blusher on the apples of your cheeks. **71**

72 You can't possibly leave the house without perfume. Dab a little of your favourite scent behind your ears – sweet.

73 Top-to-Toe Beauty – pat yourself all over with your favourite body cream. Ohhh, that's lovely.

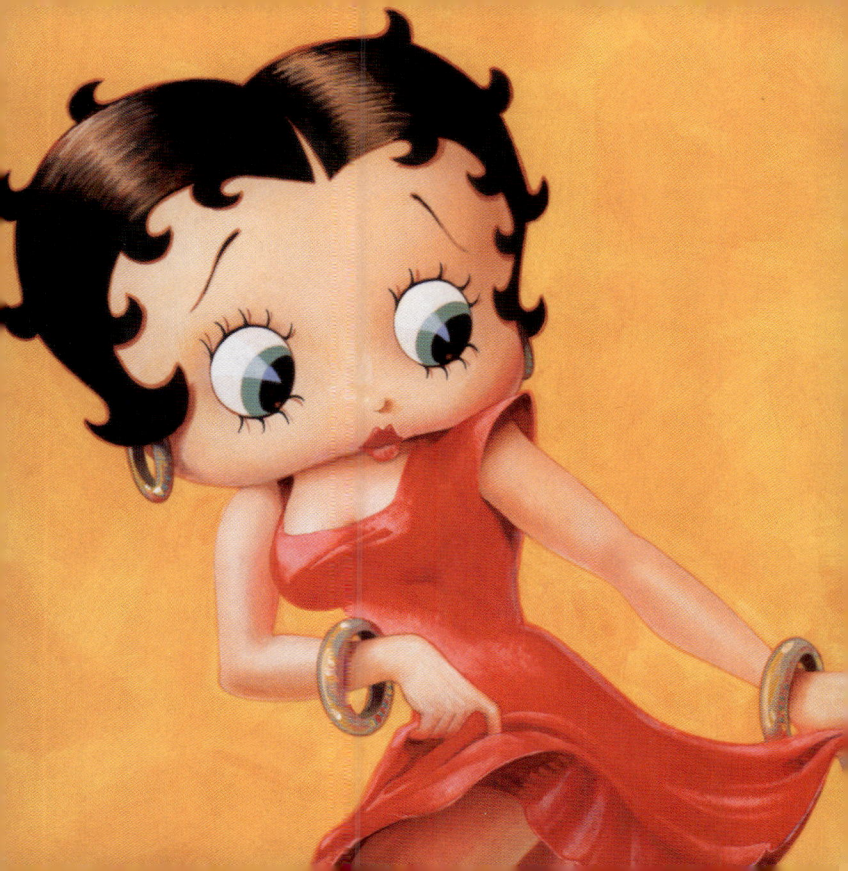

74 A facial for your feet – add a few drops of peppermint to some hot water and relax – footsie heaven!

75 The easiest way to look good is lots of sleep, lots of water, lots of exercise – Mother Nature really does know best.

76 Tan-tilize! For a glowing (and safe) tan, always fake, never bake!

77 Twist (don't plunge) that mascara wand to get more on the brush – it's easy when you know how.

78

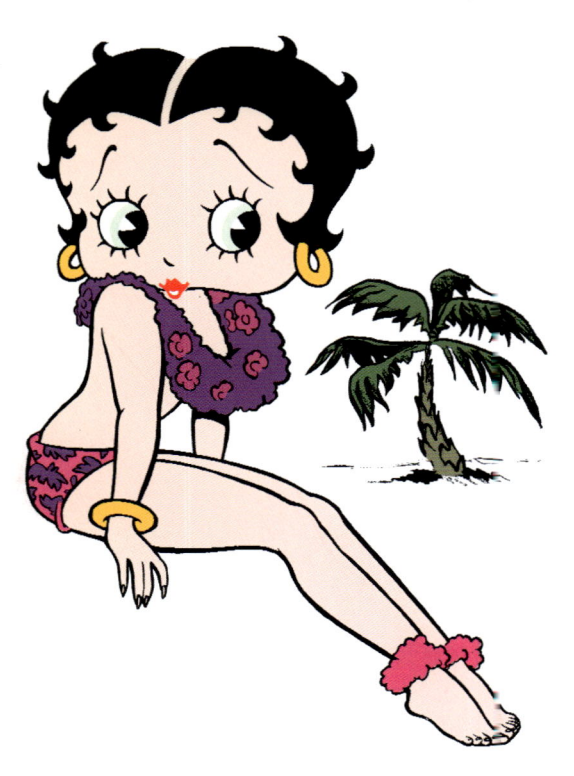

Betty Boop's boot camp says: always look beach-tastic. Waterproof mascara is my secret weapon.

79 Some say lipstick on your teeth means you're going to get kissed – some smudges we don't mind!

80 I always rub in hand cream before bed... they're so soft come morning-time.

81 If you're wearing strappies, paint your toe nails a lovely bright colour – want to paint the town red too?

82 You need to keep those legs in trim, so forget the lift and take the stairs. What a view!

83 Mirror, mirror on the wall... carry a pocket mirror, for a quick make-up fix.

84 Soft nails, oh my! To stop them splitting, file them with the polish still on.

85 Spa Boop – fluffy white robe; check, soft warm towels; check, favourite scented candle; check... the perfect home spa with a definite NO RUSH POLICY

Golden Tip – I use a little waxy lip balm to moisturise my nails – it really works! **86**

BETTY'S Beauty SALON

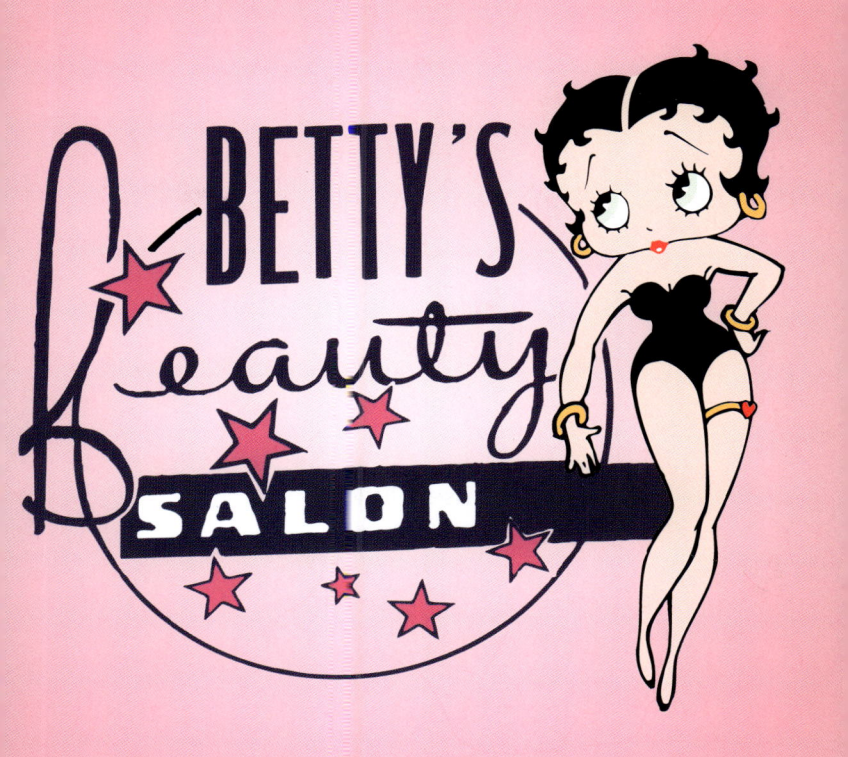

87 Protect your hands – wear gloves – even I do the dishes, sssshhh!

88 If you look good, you feel good – it's that simple! Boop-oop-a-doop!

89 Don't forget those knees, they need cream too – thank you!

90 T-A-N-T-A-S-T-I-C. Don't forget to exfoliate and moisturise before putting on fake tan – and remember to use gloves!

91 Keep your hands super soft with a little face mask – silky, smooth and scrumptious.

92

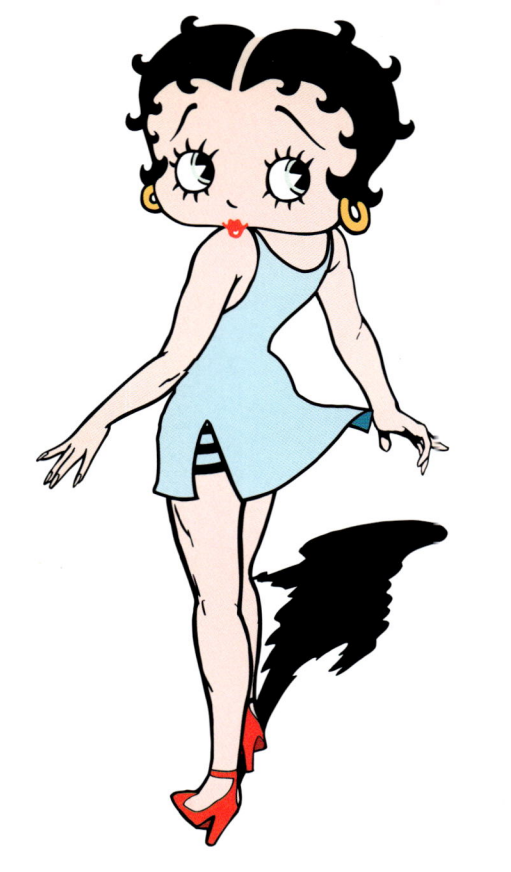

Want show-stopping legs? Dust a little shimmer powder down the centre of your shin – watch out world, I'm coming through!

93 Cuticles need a little help? Try using an orange stick after a bath or shower when they're nice and soft. It works, yes it does!

94 For tootsies like mink, soak your feet in a bowl of warm milk and sit back. Can you pass me the grapes please?

95 Try mixing your favourite fragrance with a little almond oil and rub into your arms, chest and legs – why, you really are heaven-scent.

96 Oh, are those feet aching from too much shopping? Lash on lots of cream, pop on some silky socks, and then catch up on your beauty sleep. By morning – hey, presto, super soft!

97 Nudge nudge! Keep those elbows smooth and soft with a little extra lotion.

Don't forget to exercise. **98**

99

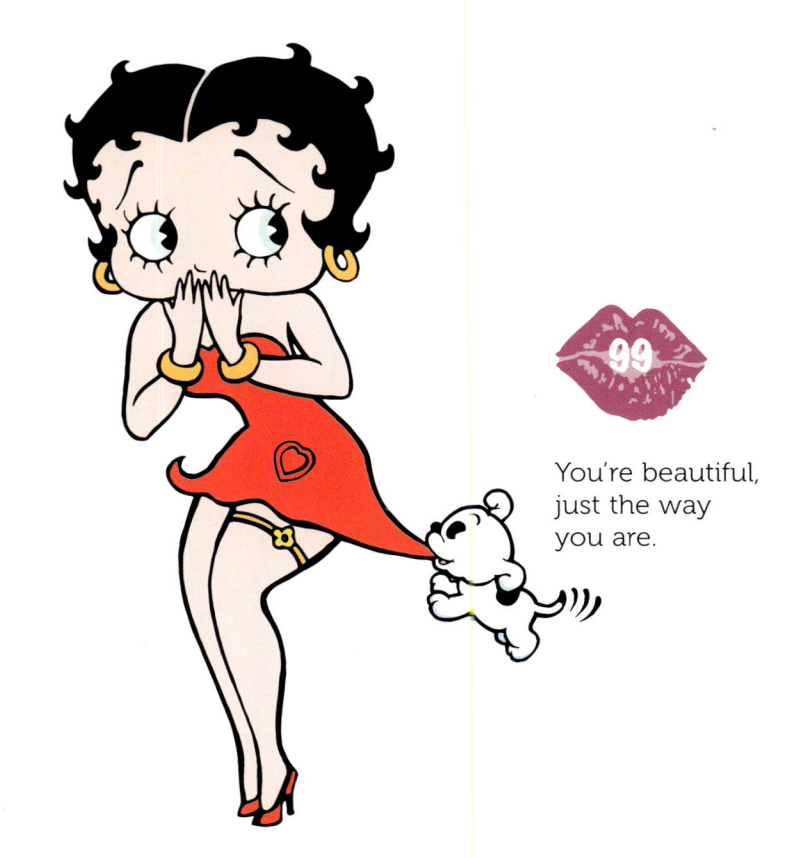

You're beautiful, just the way you are.

Love,
Betty x

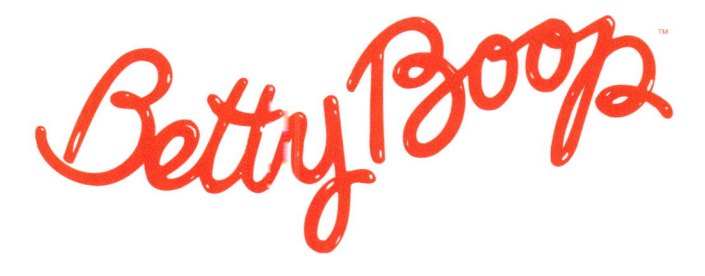

Betty Boop™

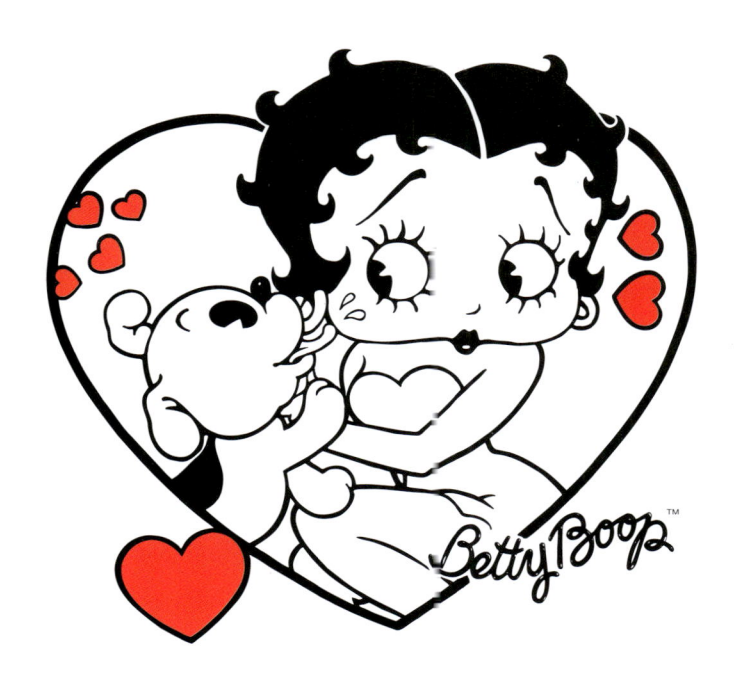

Look out for more secrets from **Betty Boop...**

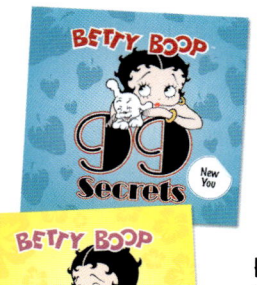

New You
We all need a boost from time to time. Miss Boop shows us lots of little things that make a very big difference. Juicy fruit drinks, sunny thoughts and healthy tips for a New You, you'll love!

Happiness
Being happy is easier than you think! Think lovely, warm, fresh towels. A cosy picnic for two. Falling in love – ahhh. Secrets to make you and everybody else happy, too!

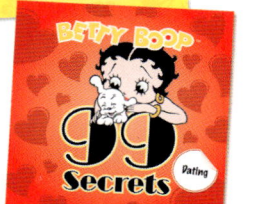

Dating
Miss Boop's tips on looking date-great! Where should you meet on a first date? Is he Prince Charming or just another frog? Betty Boop is the expert – she's here to help you get it right!

www.bettyboop.com

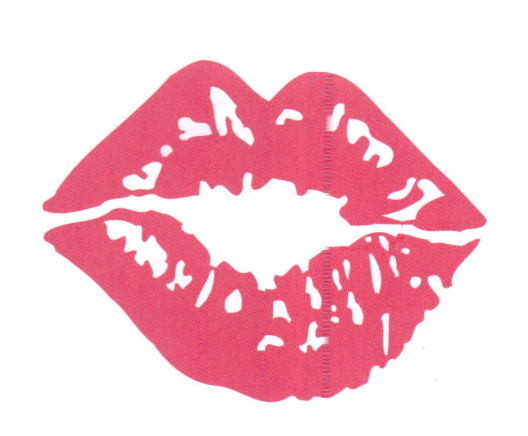

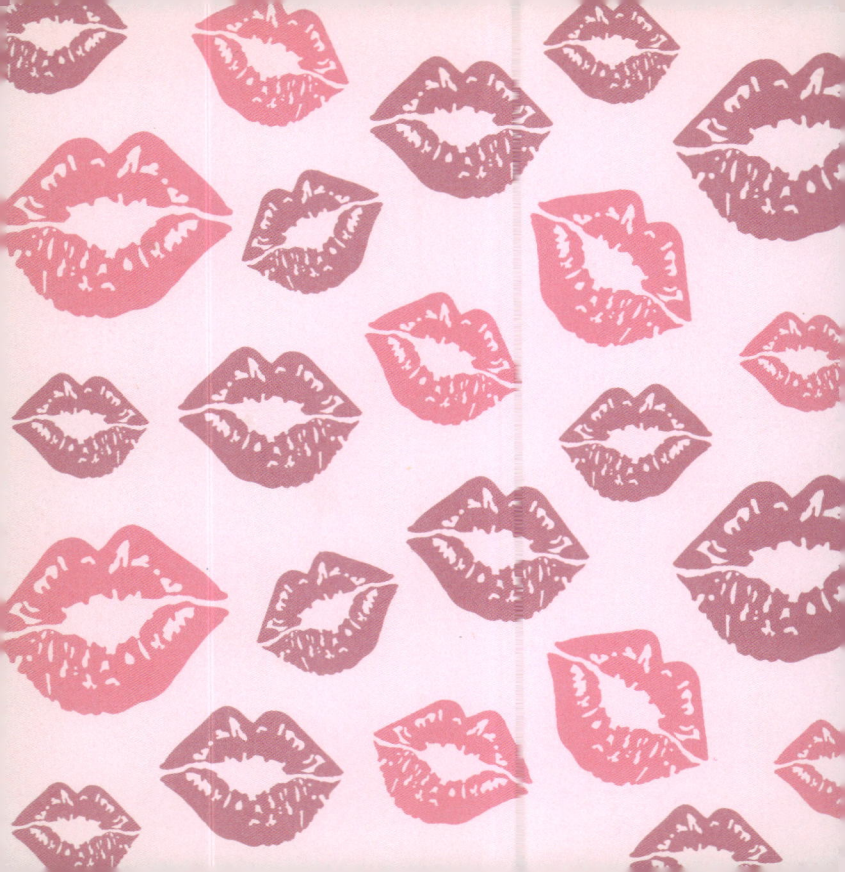